INNER GROWTH THRU REIKI

Sunny Cohen

Cover Art by Emma Wille (Suka Street Art)

Sunny Cohen Publishing

While every precaution has been taken in the preparation of this book, the publisher assumes no responsibility for errors or omissions, or for damages resulting from the use of the information contained herein.

INNER GROWTH THRU REIKI

First edition. November 29, 2023.

Copyright © 2023 Sunny Cohen.

ISBN: 979-8223778288

Written by Sunny Cohen.

Table of Contents

To the people who helped me with my recovery from MCS (Dr. Tony Esau, Dr. John Green, and Sally Green) and to those who helped me to discover Reiki (Chery Esau and Marilyn Powers). To those who encouraged me in writing this book (Kathy McCullough, Carolyn McGrath, Judy Levitow, and the late Moira Judith Mann) and to my son Jonah Saifer and daughter-in-law Jasmine Cho who've provided constant support.

Preface

As a female born in the 50s - in a home marked with alcoholism, violence, gambling addiction and infidelity - along with numerous cultural and emotional gifts, I experienced a good deal of trauma. Not only from my upbringing and the cultural currents I experienced, but later as an adult, from my own internal pressure to succeed both personally and professionally.

In my early 40s, my immune system totally broke down. I spent the years that followed engaged in a journey to reset my nervous system and regain my ability to function.

In this memoir, I discuss my early life and health breakdown, but most importantly present information about what gradually restored my physical and emotional health: Reiki, Yogic practices and involvement in the Arts. My hope is that sharing my experience will educate readers about available resources and stimulate them to take action to improve their lives.

Chapter 1

In March 2023, I felt that I received an unexpected Reiki attunement from beyond the grave.

What lies behind or progression as Reiki healers from Reiki 1 through Masters' level, in addition to our innate capacity as healers and the experience we acquire, are the attunements we receive from our instructors.

In its purest form, Reiki is a discipline that is handed down from teacher to student and is based on a bond between them. Attunements catalyze the development of the individual's ability to deliver Reiki. Each level of Reiki training features an attunement strengthening the student's connection with the Reiki energy and the ability to transmit it.

This is the story of the surprise, bonus Reiki attunement I believe I received. In March 2023, when I visited my son Jonah and his wife Jasmine in Japan, they were dedicated hosts, sharing with me all of the tourist spots in Tokyo most visitors might want to see. But as a Reiki Master and practitioner of Reiki for 25 years, I was not the typical tourist.

In the midst of our travels, I suggested to them that I would like to visit the gravesite of Dr. Mikao Usuii, the originator of contemporary Reiki. Jonah and Jasmine were very generous in not only locating the site in the Pure Land Saiho-ji Temple grounds, navigating our way there in the Tokyo suburbs, but accompanying me.

It took some doing to actually locate the Saiho-ji Temple. Once we exited the subway stop, after around 15 minutes of wandering around the picturesque streets and asking for directions, some of which were correct and many of which weren't, we finally located the grounds. Much to my relief, after knocking on a locked gate, a guard admitted us and pointed the way to Usuii's gravesite.

It was a pleasure to visit and experience the lovely gravesite, not only to reach our desired location after the search, but also because it was a sunny day and the atmosphere and the energy of the cemetery grounds was nurturing and protective.

After a little while, Jonah and Jasmine departed the cemetery plot to hang out closer to the entry of the grounds, leaving me to commune by myself with Dr. Usui's gravesite. I briefly basked in the comforting energy of my surroundings before telepathically sending a message of appreciation to Usuii, thanking him for his contribution of Reiki to the World and to Humanity. In response, to my surprise, I felt a telepathic jolt, like a full-body kick-in-the-pants, and a message in my head "It's your turn now!!!" Was that an attunement or just an admonition from beyond the grave to get cracking? Whichever it was, it fortified my commitment to my Reiki practice and to disseminate whatever wisdom I have been blessed to acquire.

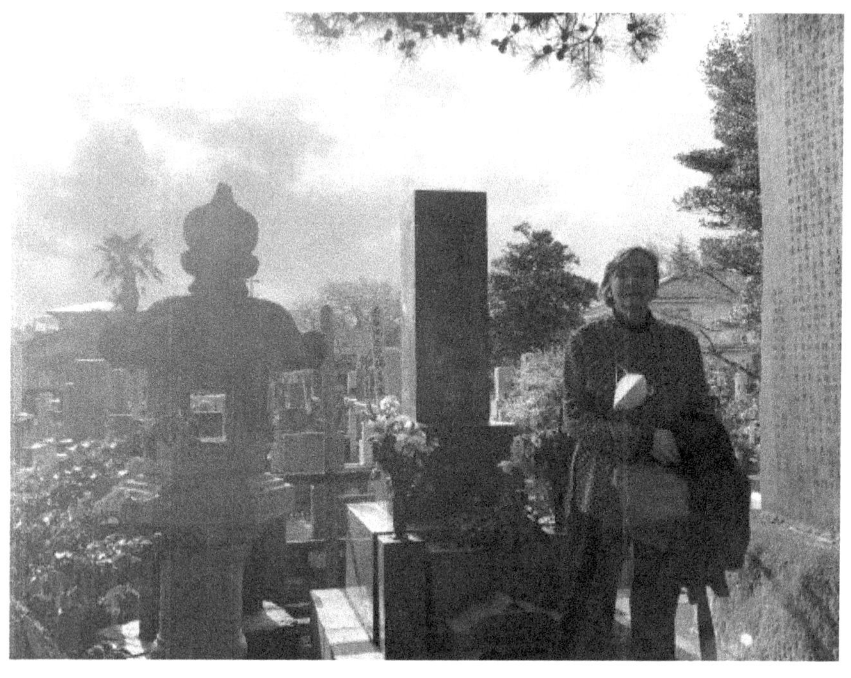

Dr. Usui's Reiki Precepts

Just for Today:

1. Don't get angry.
2. Don't worry.
3. Show appreciation.
4. Work hard (on yourself).
5. Be kind to others.

Chapter 2

Our Reiki appointment is for 2 PM here in Cuenca, Ecuador. My client is in Columbia, so thankfully there are no time zone differences to wrangle. I check in with her at 1:30 PM via Whatsapp to see how she is feeling and if any additional symptoms have cropped up since we last communicated.

She first contacted me because of feelings of hopelessness and depression. As we interacted, I learned that she had a complicated personal history and a panapoly of emotional and physical symptoms. Less than a year ago, she was struck by a truck while riding a bike in Barcelona, where she was stationed for work, rendering her arm, neck and shoulder chronically painful and near useless. Now, temporarily residing in her childhood home with her parents, she is marinating in an atmosphere of unresolved childhood issues. And suffering emotionally and physically.

She returns my Whatsapp message at 1:32, informing me that today she has a headache. But her depression has lifted since our last session several weeks ago, and she has much less pain in her shoulder, neck and arm. And she's experiencing far fewer feelings of uncontrollable anger towards her father. Overall much improved.

I conclude that the Reiki I sent her at our last session is largely responsible for her reported improvement. But as a natural skeptic, Reiki's powers for curing my clients still strains even my credibility.

Today's Reiki Session

After checking in with my client, I prepare myself for our distance Reiki session. I lie down, dim the lights, and place crystals strategically on different parts of my body. Then I turn on binaural beats music, which

I listen to with headphones. First the music puts me in a meditative state before I transition into a zone of altered consciousness to deliver Distance Reiki. I connect with my client through an intuitive feeling sense prior to becoming receptive to the visions and energies that automatically flow through me in response to her needs. I recognize that I am in the Reiki zone when I feel the energy pulsing in my hands and fingers.

Once in this altered state, I focus on my client. I think about her issues: her desire for a good husband and family, her feelings of having been dominated and suppressed while growing up, and the physical pain in her body. Pictures automatically appear in my mind's eye. I visualize my client accompanied by a kind and caring partner at a beautiful, resplendent wedding. I see her partner coming to her assistance, halting a negative interaction between herself and her father. A scenario of such images run through my mind for around 15 minutes. Then the pulsing of energy in my hands and fingers abruptly stops letting me know that our session is over: it is time to stop my active participation in her healing process.

I can never anticipate what a distance session will hold except that energy will start flowing through my hands at the appointed time and, in most cases, will reliably halt in around 15 minutes. I cannot predict what pictures – if any – will appear, what sensations I will feel as I tune into my client, or the intensity of the energy that will pulse through my hands and fingers.

I also cannot predict how the client will respond to the treatment. Some times, the client will feel nothing during the session but afterwards will feel an improvement. In other cases, the client will feel worse while receiving the Reiki energy but will ultimately feel better. And at other times the client will have a pleasant relaxing experience without noticeable results. Or any combination of these experiences. As a Reiki practitioner, I am a channel for Universal Life Force Energy, bearing neither the responsibility – nor the credit – for the healing that is usually effected. With Reiki, the practitioner delivers a session in partnership with the receiver. The healing can only be as effective as the client is capable of receiving and catalyzing for self healing.

But removing my ego is a challenge. Socialized to be a caretaker, I have had to learn to stop taking responsibility for the outcome.

My Experience as a Reiki Practitioner

I have been practicing Reiki for over 20 years, and my healing abilities have increased greatly during that time. Reiki is a spiritual practice that enables the practitioner to tune into the Universal Energetic Force Field and distribute Life Force Energy. Through participating in this practice, I have experienced the development of a personal spiritual connection along with an expansion of my intuitive abilities and an increase in self-acceptance and self-love along with the ability to self-regulate.

Recently, in addition to an increase in my skills to enact healing in people in person and over distances, to my surprise I have also experienced the ability to heal – and communicate telepathically – with animals including dogs, llamas and wild horses.

What has been the cause for the increase in my abilities, along with the normal increase in mastery that comes with over 20 years of experience and progressing from Reiki Level 1 through Reiki Master? One of my Reiki Masters, Chery Esau, recently shared with me that the present time is one in which light energy is needed to counter the dark, and many healers are experiencing a great expansion of their abilities. Additionally, my theory is that training and exposure to my excellent teacher/practitioners, Marilyn Powers and Chery Esau, both of Portland, Oregon USA and the Usui School of Reiki, have greatly benefitted me.

This book chronicles my journey in my ability to heal self and others, sharing the lessons that my journey may perhaps also hold for you.

Chapter 3

In 1992 - at the age of 40 – I found myself getting sick repeatedly. I would have one set of symptoms, for example, from the flu, and then a whole other set of symptoms would arise two weeks - or even just a week - later. This went on for several months.

My chiropractor/acupuncturist, Dr. Sally Green, referred me to a new primary care doctor known for her diagnostic abilities. During our second or third appointment she threw up her hands and let me know that she thought my main problem was being a hypochondriacal malingerer. And it wasn't like going to the doctor was all I had on my plate although it could have been – from downtown Portland, I was commuting to the Portland Silicon Valley to fulfill an instructional design contract and caring for my young son half time, shared custody.

I would learn – a lot later - that the high-tech business for which I was working was responsible for my illness. This unnamed company, now defunct, was housed in a three-building complex connected by bridges, and was not properly circulating the neurotoxins resulting from their manufacturing. The poisons were hundreds of times the level allowed by OSHA.

After a few months of revolving illnesses, my chiropractor, Sally Green, referred me to a different doctor who she said treated people who had been sick for a long time.

The visit to Dr. John Green proved to be revelatory. John Green was a specialist in environmental illness and auto-immune disease, and he pegged my problem. It was Multiple Chemical Sensitivities (MCS), also known as Environmental Illness. Over the next few months I would repeatedly make the journey to his comforting country office around an hour from Portland where I was living. I always looked forward to the light-filled drive – I sped on I5 for 30 minutes or so before exiting and meandering through bucolic Oregon small towns.

On the one hand, appointments with Dr. Green were full of information that would set me reeling: early on, he delivered the news that I had a syndrome, Multiple Chemical Sensitivities (MCS), from which I might never recover. But at the same time our interaction and his presence were comfortable and deeply reassuring. He was not a typical doctor: appointments with him were unhurried, and communication felt intimate and synergistic. I sensed that he was truly present – that he was completely there for me. That he sought to know my whole self - not just my symptoms. That I, and my wellness, were a priority to him, spurring me to make them my priority as well.

These visits were simultaneously surreal – and magical. They provided a liminal space with a spaciousness absent from my abrasive life. I was experiencing a wake-up call. My life could not continue as it had – I literally would not survive it. My interaction with Dr. Green galvanized me to make different choices to dig myself out of my predicament.

At an early appointment, I met the mayor of a neighboring town in the waiting room who I learned was recovering from the same problem; she did not present as a sick person but glowed with health and intelligence – I chose to be reassured and to take that as a sign that I too would recover.

While waiting for Dr. Green in his inner office, I read a maxim on his wall: "If I don't take care of my body, where will I live?" I had never seen this philosophy expressed by doctors I had known previously. Another indicator of Dr. John Green's spiritual – and very alternative – approach to medicine.

I went through extensive allergy tests at Dr. Green's office and learned that I had "sensitivities" to multiple foods and everyday things in the environment including oil heat, gasoline, synthetics, paint, plastics, scented products, and smoke. Dr. Green counseled me that my cure would come from removing these influences from my life as much as possible: this required paring down my diet to the skeletal number of foods that did not bother me and changing my lifestyle, replacing many items in my 1927 North Portland bungalow home. I stopped using my oil furnace and bought a number of small electric heaters. I ripped the carpets up from the floors, which fortunately were wood. I replaced my sheets, towels, and blankets with all cotton items, and found alternative cleaning and personal hygiene products.

Spending this kind of money on my self care was revolutionary. My mother, a child of the depression, had raised me to be frugal and self denying even though my parents earned an upper middle-class income. Now with a minute and precarious income, I was unquestioningly making these purchases for my self- care.

What I was going through physically, psychologically and financially was deeply unnerving. My personal support network was flimsy. I was separated from my former husband, who at least earlier in our relationship had provided most of my emotional support, and I was not close to my family. I felt deserted by most of my "friends" and became embittered by their lack of care and concern. I remember complaining to a mutual friend of a good friend who was MIA; he explained that I freaked her out because I reminded her of the abandonment she felt when her mother had cancer. I was baffled by the acceptance and matter-of-factness with which he offered this information.

Too, I was on my own financially. A few people – a friend and my brother – gave me one-time fiscal reinforcements, much appreciated. Another godsend was my husband deferring filing for divorce, allowing me to stay on his health insurance, obviously sorely needed at that time. But my financial resources were slim, so I had to keep working despite my illness.

I accepted an instructional design contract lasting for the next year or so at the Weyerhaeuser plant outside of Eugene, Oregon. This too was not good for my health - each visit involved a prolonged exposure to mill chemicals for a few days, the exact opposite of what the doctor had ordered. But the rest of the time I could work from home, and that was worth a lot in my debilitated condition. The contract was also devoid of most of the politics present in many of my past work experiences, and this psychic peace was also a blessing.

As my disease progressed, my symptoms were so bad that I could not wash the dishes or read a newspaper without experiencing neurological symptoms including confusion and weird tingles and spasms. My intelligence dropped; I easily lost 30 IQ points. It was scary, especially the prospect that I might not recover. The thought of possibly never being able to read normally again was especially unnerving.

Physically my experiences swung between odd sensations, deep fatigue, and unrelenting pain. It was a challenge to manage my discomfort – and my emotions. I learned new techniques for managing the pain– it usually worked to stay present and breathe thru the pangs until they dissipated.

But life was not only filled with despair. There were happy notes too. Being less intelligent was not all bad – I welcomed the decrease in neurosis that accompanied my less agile mind. I also had one old friend, Valerie Brooks, who did not desert me and was always up for a chat and attending musical events. Music captivates me; my love for music would provide solace not only at that difficult time but would reliably relieve my maladies and lift me to a higher vibration into the future too. And I found the two Dr. Greens inspiring not only in their kindness to me, but also in their examples of a way to live in the world that was based on love and integrity. I saw them as living saints. So much in the life I had inhabited in the Corporate world had been disillusioning: competitive, narrowly focused and uncaring. The Dr. Greens embodied a way of living that was consistent with my values and buttressed my will to live.

And there was a new understanding I came to about myself: I was amazed by my fierce will to survive. Over the next several years I poured all my focus into the restoration of my wellness. My unrelenting survival instinct surprised me – the lengths I would go to improve my health. Prior to getting sick, I had been working on a documentary film for over 6 years that consumed all of my focus. When it was complete, I was bereft. Recovering from Multiple Chemical Sensitivities (MCS) replaced my documentary film as the lodestar of my existence.

Chapter 4

So now it is probably an appropriate time for me to tell you more about who I am and my history.

I was born in 1952 to parent who were both (1) highly intelligent and (2) the children of Eastern European Immigrants. And they were both *Characters*, with a Capital C. Their parents - my grandparents - escaped World War 2 and the Holocaust by a relatively wide margin, fleeing pogroms for New York City in the early part of the 20th century.

Except the holocaust across the ocean still figured prominently in my father's early life. His mother and father, sweatshop workers and activists at the time, as well as Orthodox Jews, devoted every spare hour and penny to rescuing even distant family and shared their home with them once they arrived in the USA. So total was their focus that there was no economic margin for even the basics of the American Dream. My Dad told me achingly – 20 years later - how he had not even been allowed to keep a bicycle that he won at school: it had to be sold, its value converted to the transport – and rescue from annihilation - of unknown relatives.

I never really got to know well the grandparents on my father's side. We would go to visit them a time or two a year when my grandmother would serve us an elaborate traditional meal that she had spent hours preparing. Like a dignified servant, she never sat with us at the table but traversed between kitchen and dining room serving multiple courses – observing a home-based Sabbath liturgy. She would steal 5 minutes during these evenings to whisk me way to her secret chambers where she would kiss my hands, lovingly call me her "shayna maidele", and proffer a small and radiant gift from a hidden drawer. There was something shining and nourishing in those brief luminous interludes – a glimpse of the living Shekinah? My grandmother always left me wanting more of her, but even as a young girl I accepted that she gave me what she could spare.

Since her death when I was in college - I don't think anyone even suggested that I would return from the West Coast to attend her funeral – I have been looking for my Grandma Sarah in far-flung places. I even went a few years ago to the Ukraine to the site of her early life, then classified as Romania. While I gained some insight into what she saw as a young girl in the near ghost town with its view of the Carpathians, I did not find remnants of her luminosity anywhere.

My father had a conflicted relationship with her. Sarah was his father's second wife. My grandfather brought into this second marriage his developmentally disabled daughter from his previous marriage. As a teenager, my father experimented sexually with this older half sister. My father never forgave his mother for how she responded when she discovered this transgression: sending the sister away to a home. His sister was effectively banished – they never saw her again. My father recognized the injustice in this; his sister was the one castigated for what he had initiated. Later he searched for her in multiple New Jersey homes for the developmentally disabled but never found her. This is just occurring to me as I write this: was he too searching for the luminosity of a dearly loved, but hardly known, female relative?

My father fled the demands and rigors of his Orthodox Jewish home at an early age, joining the USA army in South Korea, pre-Korean War. His defective feet gave him a pass to leave his tour of duty early and take advantage of the GI Bill to start studies at New York's City College. He dreamt of being a medical doctor and poet in his spare time, a kind of Jewish Wallace Stevens. But he was diverted from his dreams in his short life of 52 years. One of the first detours was meeting and marrying my mother when he was 20 and she was 18.

My mother was also the daughter of Eastern European Jewish immigrants, but non-observant. Their religion, if they had one, was based on bagels. My mother's mother, my Grandma Mura, immigrated in her early-teens, and though highly intelligent had no formal schooling either in Poland or upon arrival to the USA. I was born when she was 50, and during our time together, she struggled mightily with arthritis, abstaining from her favorite foods and beverages to control the pain. I promised I would become a doctor in order to cure her; this pledge gladdened her. She enthralled me with tales of her life in Poland including sneaking to the top of the village schoolhouse to listen to the classes from which she, as a girl, was barred.

Throughout her life, Grandma Mura had been saddled with indignities because of her gender. Her mother, my deceased Great Grandma Elke - a larger-than-life figure I knew only by reputation—always preferred Grandma's older brother, Bobby, and showed it in a multitude of ways. Yet living with her mother throughout her life, Mura contorted herself to withstand Elke's domination. Grandma Mura confided in me how glad she was to take control of her own kitchen after Elke passed away.

Elke favored my mother – not unusual in grandparent/grandchild relationships –and still my mother felt neglected. A child of the depression, she envied Shirley Temple and wondered why her family directed so much adoration towards the child star while ignoring her - the child star in their midst.

My mother could have been considered brilliant - she came in second statewide on a high school New York State Math standardized test. Like my father, she had unfulfilled dreams. An animal lover, as a girl her desire was to become a veterinarian. But she was unable to gain entry to the Pre-vet program at City College - there were limits to the sizes of the classes and attempting to bend the rules did not occur to her - so she could not prepare for the veterinary profession.

My mother, too, married early to escape from the home life that she found restrictive and oppressive. Like my father, she eventually came to find their marriage had propelled her into a nightmare rather than her dreams. As a young corporation executive, my father began womanizing while my mother was isolated in suburbia where they moved to support his career. By their divorce in 1963, when he left her and our family to marry another woman, she had become a full-fledged alcoholic.

In our secular household, no one ever taught me how to pray. My parents reveled in their atheism. I still recall an incident during my childhood that chilled me to my core. I was three or four when I asked my parents what happens after death. Glancing askance to seek my father's approval, which he magnanimously conferred, my mother glibly answered that humans were deposited into the ground. With disbelief I asked if people stay there forever. They cheerfully agreed from the front seat of the car. The sky took on an eerie cast for the remainder of our evening journey. I reeled from the prospect of this horrible fate for a long time after that. My parents' lack of ability to attend to my spiritual needs affected me deeply.

On several occasions, late at night and alone in my bedroom, when I was around the same age, I saw groupings of translucent figures. They were oblivious to my presence and absorbed in activity. I was puzzled by the identity of these beings but now realize that what I saw were ghosts.

Somehow by the age of 7, I knew how to "cast spells", which I did frequently with the intent of keeping my parents' increasingly frayed union together through the loud arguments and whispered infidelities. Until one day, after too many midnight bathroom encounters with the dog shivering from the intensity of my parents' fights, I decided their marriage was not worth saving and ceased my efforts. As I was not certain of my powers, I did not know whether to be surprised or not when they split soon after.

My early environment was one in which family torment was fomenting. As a young child I was my mother's rock – without much other support she relied on me to support her emotionally, and to take an active role – far beyond my years – to try to stem the conflict in her marriage.

I remember being woken at an early age – maybe 5 or 6 – to the sight of my father leaving the house with a packed suitcase. "Your father is leaving", my mother shouted through tears. "Get him to stay", she beseeched. I cannot remember what I did, but whatever it was, it resulted in the extension of their miserable marriage.

Being Mother's Little Helper gave me a kind of power in the domestic universe. At times I felt that in my mother's eyes I was so much more substantial than my father, who was alternatively violent and betraying, and my baby brother who filled the house with his colicky cries and otherwise seemed to contribute little. Addicted to my mother's approval, I would seek to help her in any way she asked – from taking charge of the house; to babysitting, though terrified, on mid-week "date nights" when no babysitter was available. Through a telepathic link to my mother and my connection to another realm, I would also find her lost keys and glasses – I received pictures in my minds eye of where the items were located. And my inborn knowledge of how – and when – to cast spells often resulted in what I was petitioning for, usually on behalf on others rather than myself.

But in the outside world, as a young child, overweight and without social skills, I was a misfit and target for bullies. As the years went on, and I acquired friends and some confidence in my own abilities, the lure of my peers and the world outside my home grew stronger as the domestic sphere disintegrated. What was left in our home was an alcoholic mother and in a large colonial house on the other side of town – where we had to spend alternate weekends – a defensive, angry and alienating father who had adopted a waspy wife and a white bread life in his eagerness to assimilate.

Could I be blamed for this turn of events since I had turned away from my intuitive gifts, no longer casting spells or finding lost objects for my mother? My mother's alcoholism blurred the telepathic bond we once shared. I had ceased pouring my emotional energy into the preservation of our doomed family. I closed the door on my psychic abilities, glad to exchange them for what seemed like success in the outside world and the social realm.

Chapter 5

Fast Forward: 1992

It's been 28 years since I shut down my intuitive gifts at the age of 12. Grandma Mura died around that time, my parent's marriage *finally* broke up, and my mother became a full-blown alcoholic. This was the 60s in New York City, where we had moved, and my mother's drinking propelled me onto an independent path as a free-spirited teenaged female worshipping in the Church of Sex, Drugs, and Rock 'n Roll.

In my years of adolescence and young adulthood, although I pursued astrology and metaphysics, my intuitive skills became a thing of the past that I rarely thought of revisiting. During college, at a metaphysical bookstore in Portland that I frequented, I asked the owners if they recommended developing my psychic abilities. They warned me against it, saying that it would be disruptive and would ruin my life with unpleasant knowledge about random people I would encounter. Ambivalent – and busy with other concerns - I let the matter of reconnecting to my intuitive abilities drop after that and did not think about it again for a long time. Only in recent years has my intuition reemerged, but in a way that supports me and others; connected with Reiki, it is not destructive, thankfully contradicting the store owners' prediction.

The artistic activity that I loved – and fit in when I could - was an intuitive practice too although I did not recognize it then as such. When acting as a theater writer and director starting in college and lasting for the next 7 or so years, I found myself embodied in the present. These experiences were luminous, an unusual sensation; I usually felt awkward, even depressed, and disconnected from my body. I now understand that the spiritual connection is much of what has drawn me to creative practices. I later would find this to be true as a filmmaker and also as a lyricist. I realize now that there is something about artistic processes that allow the channeling of knowledge and messages from other dimensions.

But although being a performing and moving image artist was what set me on fire, making me feel like my true self, I spent much of my early life torn between creative pursuits and "fitting in", achieving, and surviving monetarily: as a wife and mother and as a professional worker. The messages from my Jewish mother and from my social world to marry and procreate were strong, and the man I married – though, ironically, we met when working in a theater – was only supportive of my artistic activities and fulfillment in a limited way. He claimed to be a feminist, as did my mother, but both my husband and mother echoed the oppressive demands of an unequal world. And I was conflicted – I wanted to please them and was not yet strong enough to claim what I needed for myself except surreptitiously. As the child of an alcoholic, I had been conditioned to be a people pleaser. (At 70, I am finally learning to loosen those shackles.)

Until at the age of 38, serious illness halted me in my tracks, causing me to enter a long period of healing which ultimately called forth once again my intuitive self. This mysterious illness took months to unravel and identify. And over 10 years to recover from.

The illness had been preceded not only by the breakup of my marriage but also by finishing a documentary film that had taken over 6 years to complete. Due to a lack of funding, it required months of inadequate sleep for its completion. Post production services were supplied by a local PBS Station and took place from 11 PM to 5 in the morning.

The emptiness I felt in the dissolution of my marital relationship of 14 years broke my heart. It had become clear that we were not compatible enough for the long haul, but we were family - and at one time had been very close.

Even more painful was the adjustment of sharing custody and only seeing my young son part time.

As for the film, it was a huge letdown to be left in an impoverished situation after years of dedication. The film won critical accolades and awards: a 5 star review in *Library Journal*, PBS showings, and a Bronze Apple in the National Educational Film and Video Festival among other distinctions. I achieved some moments of glory but not much else besides a few glowing reviews and incandescent memories. In the aftermath of these experiences, after several months of delivering pizza, I returned to my corporate profession and did a training contract at a high-tech company where I was exposed to a high level of neurotoxins, damaging my already stressed immune system.

What followed were five tumultuous years: of discovering what my illness actually was and doing everything possible to recover.

Chapter 6

I can separate my recovery roughly into two distinct phases. What I will call *Phase 1* lasted for approximately five years. During that time I experienced acute symptoms and wondered at least once a day if I would actually ever recover. Because of my inability to tolerate the exposures in the everyday world, I was distinctly limited in my ability to live a normal life, to go to my usual places and engage in my routine activities. Life – and the world - took on a surreal hue.

In *Phase 2,* which lasted for the next four years, my symptoms decreased substantially due to my recovery. I was able to emerge into the regular world but still had to constantly monitor my well-being, conscious of my reactions to food and exposures in my environment.

Throughout this entire 9-year period, environmental illness dominated my life. I endeavored to engage in activities to improve not only my physical health but also my mindset. Somewhere in the midst of working with Dr. John Green, I had come to perceive environmental illness as a psycho-spiritual malady, and I knew I had to address my psychological frailties in addition to the more mundane physical ones. I had grown up in many ways neglected in an alcoholic, and sometimes violent, home – so it made sense that I had some psychological weaknesses. I came to understand that my disease had a psychological component: it was a two-fold problem involving boundaries – (1) feeling that my boundaries were inadequate and (2) that they were encroached upon.

Phase 1 of Recovery

I wrote earlier about discovering my illness and my work with Dr. John Green, who first diagnosed me. Around a year into Phase 1, I made a discovery that stunned me - other patients of Dr. Green's had - like me

- been workers at the same high-tech company: we had all become ill as a result of working there. This un-named Beaverton, Oregon high tech manufacturing company consisted of three connected buildings, and it turned out that it had not been properly ventilated; the neurotoxins were hundreds of times the amount allowed by OSHA.

While I initially entertained the thought of suing, a lawyer friend advised me against it. He told me that it was close to impossible to prevail in class action suits in Oregon and that going to court with my own lawsuit would expose me to humiliating personal attacks. He suggested that it would be better to commit to my recovery and avoid the psychological distress inherent in the legal route.

Several of Dr. Green's patients pursued successful lawsuits, but they had been fulltime workers and had accepted their disability as permanent, wanting to be compensated for what they had undergone and future losses. I had only completed a 6-week contract, not all of it onsite, and had not accepted my illness as permanent. I was desperately trying to recover my health!

Instead of suing, I committed myself to learning everything I could about the illness. My objective was to produce a documentary to communicate everything I was learning about environmental injury. I found the topic of environmental illness - a twilight, but pervasive, public health issue - to be an intellectually and emotionally fertile one. I learned that there were victims of chemical injury in many spheres – former hairdressers, construction workers, office staff in sick buildings, educators in improperly built trailers without adequate ventilation (not to mention their students), military personnel exposed to chemical warfare including substances like Agent Orange. Toxic exposures were seemingly everywhere. I communicated with - and learned the heart-breaking stories of - so many people who were now living half-lives because of their chemical injuries. Speaking to these people and reading voluminous materials confirmed my surreal experience; pursuing my curiosity helped to ease my anxiety.

As I learned more, I became convinced that a major contributor to environmental illness was the lack of testing of combinations of chemicals. While my deep dive took place nearly 30 years ago, I have learned that more recent research about endocrine-disrupting chemicals (in the year 2020) confirms my hypothesis.

I took beginning steps towards making the documentary, but was not able to garner the support required to complete it. This was a controversial subject and difficult to get funded, unlike my previous documentary about auctioneering in rural America, for which I had received funding from the National Endowment for the Arts among other donors. Despite its lack of appeal to mainstream funders, this research about chemical injury was a life-giving activity for me.

My research also prepared me later on, as I regained my health, to do some video production contracts for government organizations related to this topic. At a conference whose videotapes I produced for the Agency for Toxic Substances and Disease Registry (ATSDR) in Washington DC, I had the opportunity to meet – and interview – Theron Randolph (now deceased), the doctor who discovered Multiple Chemical Sensitivity, also known as the Environmental Illness syndrome. I was truly touched and exhilarated to be in his presence! It felt like the culmination of my research - and wellness – journey to have the honor of interacting with this hero.

Also around a year or so into my illness, I began treatment with a new doctor, a naturopathic physician, Dr. Anthony Esau of the Parkrose Naturopathic Clinic. He, too, was recommended by my Chiropractor/ Acupuncturist Dr. Sally Green. While Dr. John Green had been a godsend in identifying my illness and giving me practices to keep it from progressing, Tony had the knowledge, skills and remedies to actually restore me to health. An outlier in the USA, Tony uses a machine - commonly used by MDs in Europe - that specifically diagnoses physical ailments and the medicines to treat them by connecting to a patient's acupuncture points. Tony collaborated with physicians in Germany, from where he imported his medicines. For a number of years, I had appointments with Tony a few times a month. I would sit in his homespun office, decorated with fighter planes, in an industrial part of North East Portland while Tony hooked me up to his machine and explained the significance of the displays on the computer screen. And made curative remedies for me to ingest until the next appointment.

Tony's care put me on the road to recovery. My physical limits expanded, and I could start doing new things. I would work with Tony for many years to come, and he and his wife Chery became dear friends – and in the future, Chery would teach me Reiki 2 and eventually anoint me as a Reiki Master.

I also joined a yoga group called the Art of Living that utilized a breathing practice, Sudarshan Kriya Yoga, as well as meditation techniques. We followed the teachings and techniques of Sri Sri Ravi Shankar, an Indian guru. Participating in this group, I made friends with a number of compatible people, benefitted from the camaraderie and the physical and psychological benefits of the breathing practice, and – importantly through the teachings of Shankar - overcame my crippling fear of death.

Another activity that brought healing – and inspiration - was joining a gospel choir. My friend, Marsha, a former co-worker from 10 years prior, invited me to a concert her choir was giving when I happened to run into her some place in town. It was a very welcome invitation since - due to my current intolerance of cigarette smoke - I could no longer go to musical performances at bars. I had a blast at the concert, hearing music that made my heart soar - and I, along with the other audience members, were encouraged to join in! Seeing that I took to the experience like a duck to water, Marsha invited me to join the choir. I gratefully accepted. The choir met once a week at the neighborhood African American Episcopal Church and performed every Sunday at church. Too, we often met up with other city gospel choirs to give concerts during the weekends and at public venues during the holidays. The choir members made me feel included although I was the only white person who participated.

Singing in the gospel choir was elevating on a number of levels. Being surrounded by the uplifting melodies and the vocal artistry of the choir members as we rehearsed and performed strengthened and exhilarated me. Although not a Christian, and still exploring my religious identity, I found meaning in – and was touched by - the minister's sermons. I was heartened by the authenticity of the churchgoers, inspired by their faith. And I was cheered by the spirit and kindness of the other choir members. I appreciated being part of this group and the love, support, humor and cooperation they shared, often lacking in mainstream white society. I concluded that this loving subculture is what enables many African Americans to tolerate the indignities and harshness they encounter in the outside world.

Additionally, my choir colleagues expressed the mindset that God was accountable for an individual singer's performance, relieving the individual singer of responsibility for good and bad performances. As I had sung all my life but suffered from disabling stage fright, adopting this point of view brought me substantial relief. I was able to start doing my share of solos, without the self-consciousness that had previously plagued me.

Phase 2 of Recovery

Continuing these pursuits, particularly the medical treatment of Dr. Tony Esau who addressed any physical problems as they arose, I gradually improved. (But I was not yet entirely out of the woods as I am not almost 30 years later – construction materials can still set me off.) I was able to greatly expand my activities and movement into the world.

I continued with the Art of Living Yoga organization, and was able to travel to attend a silent meditation conference out of state.

I also worked with a gifted psychic and Rapid Eye Therapy practitioner Claudia Harrington who was able to alleviate some of my trauma. I went through several Rapid Eye Therapy sessions with her, and she taught me some very helpful visualization techniques to address various conundrums.

I also progressed in my vocal career and took a few voice lessons with jazz singer Suzi Stern while I continued with the gospel choir. Suzi encouraged me to branch out and to start singing at the jazz jams that took place regularly in Portland. This was a stretch for me. Although I had been singing for most of my life, jazz was a different genre altogether than the show music, folk music and classical music that had formed my musical foundation. I had heard jazz and loved much of what I had heard, but it was still a big leap to try to integrate the rhythm, syncopation, phrasing, and flat tones commonly used in jazz into my own vocalizations. Then there was my stage fright to contend with, somewhat alleviated by the philosophy I had picked up with the gospel choir but far from gone.

Still I pushed myself to attend a weekly jam session in my neighborhood that took place on Sunday afternoons at a venue called Steen's Coffee House. This coffee house was owned by jazz drummer Ron Steen, who programmed jazz offerings at the venue and led the weekly jam session. Despite the combination of dread and adrenaline I would feel at the prospect of performing, this event definitely had its attractions for me.

I felt simultaneously encouraged and denigrated by Steen's treatment of me as a newbie jazz singer. He scoffed at my inability to deal skillfully with the mic. He would often interrupt me in my delivery of my song, signaling to the pianist to take it from the chorus the second time through. But I really loved the music and enjoyed the festive atmosphere of the gatherings along with the friendliness and encouragement of many of the other performers. And I got a sense of accomplishment from getting up and performing my songs, from battling the stage fright and delivering a performance that some might find value in, even if it was just the song and not my rendition of it that the audience enjoyed.

Jazz became my new domain to devote myself to. The gospel choir had disbanded, and – due to lack of financial support - I had let go of my dream of doing the documentary about environmental illness. With jazz there were always new wonderful songs to dive into and new techniques to master - without the big bucks required for filmmaking. It was overcast and gloomy in Portland for more than 6 months of the year, and going to a weekly jam was a good way to dispel the sadness that could set in otherwise. I met a number of people who encouraged me in my vocalizing – from Pro's to newbies - and was invited to participate in a number of music get-togethers and gigs.

Armonica was a jazz singer who started vocalizing at the jams at around the same time as I did, and she shared the same kind of passion for the music. At the time we met, she was a District Attorney for the State of Oregon and her work required her to commute to Salem, an hour away from Portland. She had managed to commandeer her own performing slot at Steen's from 3 – 5 on Thursdays, and invited me to share the gig, taking the first hour for which she could not get back from her job in time. I gratefully accepted the opportunity, but as a fledgling jazz vocalist there were two complications: (1) finding musicians to accompany me for no pay and (2) attracting an audience and keeping them entertained. There were a lot of excellent musicians in Portland who loved to play, so finding accompanists was usually not a problem. However, I was still gaining mastery as a vocalist, and giving an inspiring performance for an hour weekly was a challenge – not to mention getting an audience in the door.

Patty Duke, who I had met at the Art of Living, was a close friend who had been steeped in metaphysics and intuitive practices for a long time. She had a friend who was a Reiki Master who was visiting Portland. She thought that adding Reiki to my singing might make my performances more compelling and suggested that I study Reiki to add an element of healing to my performances. I took Patty's advice and signed up for the weekend class.

Chapter 7

I wasn't sure what to expect when I set off for the Reiki I class that Saturday morning. I didn't know much about Reiki before starting the class – hadn't even experienced a session yet myself. I chose to go based on my fervent wish to become a more appealing performing vocalist – and trust in my friend Patty Duke's suggestion that this could be accomplished by learning Reiki.

I had prepared for our Reiki 1 training weekend by abstaining from alcohol and meat for a week as instructed. As I arrived at the meeting place for our class, I sensed that I was entering a liminal space. The environment was commonplace on the surface; the most significant part of what would take place would occur on unseen levels. Our instructor, a man in his late fifties, or early 60's, embodied to me the title of "Reiki Master", humble yet commanding, and expert about, and highly experienced in, delivering Reiki. Committed to sharing his knowledge but formal, keeping distance from the two of us in his class. With a Master's degree under my belt and the college and corporate classes and metaphysical workshops I had attended - and developed and presented - in my career as a college teacher and instructional designer, I was no stranger to schooling – academic and informal. I found this class less collegial and friendly than much of what I had experienced. But our teacher was committed to delivering a bio-spiritual curriculum, not to fuzzy feelings or interpersonal sharing.

I wondered about the other student and how she came to be there. I was in my late forties by this point, but she seemed to be in her early 20s, conventionally pretty, and "normal", someone who could fit easily into mainstream society. She didn't give the impression of someone who would be attracted to the esoteric. I never learned more about her, but I suspended my questions and judgment and was glad to be in her pleasant company for the remainder of the class.

To start, the Reiki Master instructed us in the history of how Reiki was rediscovered from the Ancient Tibetans by Japanese religious scholar and practitioner Mikao Usui, how it was transmitted to his disciple Dr. Hiyashi, and then how it was brought to the West by Mrs. Takata in 1938. Mrs. Takata was a desperately ill Hawaiian woman who went to Japan to be treated by Dr. Hiyashi and emerged, healed, to bring Reiki to the USA and an expanding number of practitioners. These historical teachings communicated our instructor's – and by extension our - lineage of Reiki practitioners.

The Master shared the Ethical Principles of Reiki developed and transmitted by Usui and adapted for contemporary use: "Just for today do not worry, Just for today do not anger, Honor your parents, teachers and elders. Earn your living honestly. Show gratitude to everything."

Then the Reiki Master transmitted the rudiments of the practice of Reiki: the hand positions and places in the body to which they should be applied, the meaning of the chakras, and how to protect oneself spiritually when delivering Reiki.

When we returned to the class after lunch break we took turns practicing on each other. Each session took around an hour. An inexplicable smell of jasmine permeated our practice, ethereal and unmistakable. I interpreted this fragrance as a sign that something was occurring that was sacred and real, although not visible. Our Master then introduced the first-degree Reiki symbols and had us practice drawing them and meditating upon them.

To end the day, our Reiki Master delivered to us the first level of initiation connecting us to the Reiki source, the Reiki 1 attunement, making it possible to distribute Reiki energy.

Little did I know at the time the spiritual healing being catalyzed in me by my participation in this weekend and the prominent place that Reiki would come to occupy in my life.

Chapter 8

Since you, my reader, might have more questions about Reiki, this chapter contains the answers to common inquiries.

What is Reiki?

Reiki is a spiritual healing practice that helps to return its recipients to balance on physical, mental, emotional, and spiritual levels. Reiki supports well-being and strengthens the individual's natural ability to self heal and to heal others. Reiki usually brings rapid stress reduction and relief from pain and anxiety.

How is Reiki Delivered and Why Does it Work?

Reiki is given through light touch - or hands above – specific locations on the body. Expert practitioners can also deliver Reiki via distance. Reiki practitioners can transmit this healing energy because they are connected to the Reiki Source through their training. The initiation process accelerates through the levels from Reiki 1 to Master Practitioner. I obtained Master Level certification in 2011, over 10 years after taking my first Reiki 1 class.

What is a Typical Reiki Session Like and What are Its Results?

Pamela Miles, author of the book *Reiki,* (Penguin Publishing Group, Kindle Edition) describes a typical Reiki session in this way: "The hands of a trained Reiki practitioner are placed lightly on a fully clothed recipient who reclines or sits comfortably. When Reiki is offered to someone who is conscious, both practitioner and recipient quickly notice a gentle shift toward relaxation. Breathing becomes slower and more comfortable, and the person may sigh or even snore as the state of relaxation deepens.

The experience of Reiki treatment is very subjective and varies from person to person and treatment to treatment. Some recipients feel a warm tingling where Reiki hands are placed, others feel soft waves of subtle pulsations flowing throughout their bodies, and others feel nothing in particular—nothing, except they are very relaxed afterward, with an enhanced sense of well-being. If the person came for treatment with pain, it usually disappears or diminishes during the session. After treatment, the recipient typically feels centered and in touch with himself in a way that is very natural, but too rarely experienced by adults living a frantic postmodern lifestyle. The sense of well-being lingers, and people frequently report an immediate improvement in sleep.

Your actual experience of Reiki may center on physical, mental, or emotional changes—a sense of relaxation, relief from pain, greater clarity, a gradual lessening of anxiety or expectations or other worrisome thoughts. Meanwhile, something far subtler is happening in the background. Very gently, very quietly, very gradually, Reiki opens an inner spiritual connection that can significantly change the way a person experiences life, a sense of connectedness that can help transform negative attitudes and create a sense of meaning and purpose. "

What is the Evidence for Reiki's Effectiveness?

Miles reports that studies have found Reiki to be associated with:

• Decreased levels of stress • improvement in immune function • remedied blood pressure • Self reported lessening of anxiety, pain, and fatigue • lowered heart rate • better mood and functioning in depressed patients • overall enhanced well-being and increased vitality...

Miles also writes that the many populations that are thought to benefit from Reiki are some of those whom medical science considers hardest to treat—"those with fibromyalgia and AIDS, and victims of heart attacks. The benefits of Reiki can—and are—being delivered in the most stressful of settings—the cardiac-care unit, the delivery room, the operating room, intensive-care units, and the emergency room."

Research in Reiki's effectiveness is continuing to aggregate, with solid Scientific evidence accumulating of its efficacy.

Chapter 9

The following Thursday at Steen's Coffeehouse, I eagerly gauged the reaction of the small audience. Did the acquisition of Reiki 1 help to improve the reception of my performance? I did not detect anything. As usual, people were alternately engaged in the music and equally immersed in conversation with their tablemates. My audience did not appear to be "wowed". Patty's prescription had not worked, at least not yet.

For many months, the rest of my life proceeded as usual. Aside from performing and bringing up my adolescent son half time, I was working and commuting, contracting as an instructional designer at Intel Corporation. And for fun, attending jazz at the many live music spots around Portland and practicing with friendly musicians when I got the chance. I did not perceive anything occurring that was out of the ordinary or different than my life pre-Reiki.

Then one day, I happened to be talking with Chery, my naturopath Tony Esau's wife, when she was filling in as his receptionist. I had not realized that Chery, a nurse, was a Reiki Master and that Tony, too, had expertise in Reiki. I confided in Chery that I had done the beginning Reiki weekend training, but my practice since then had been dormant. Chery shared her opinion that I needed additional resources to continue on my Reiki Path. She offered to do a trade with me to reactivate my practice. Chery's feedback about my performance reminded me of some technical points I had forgotten and gave me confidence in my abilities. The Reiki she shared touched me profoundly with the comforting and subtle power of its energy.

Chery encouraged me to practice at every opportunity, and that's what I proceeded to do over the next few years. Often when I became aware that someone in my presence was suffering with a physical ailment, I would offer to give them some Reiki, no charge. It was always a surprise – and a rush! - to be able to alleviate the pain of a friend or stranger who was suffering.

The first time this occurred, I worked on a young Black child on a playground who was complaining of a neck ache. After gaining permission from his guardian, I asked him to relax, instructing him to breathe deeply. Then I put my hands over the spot on his body that was hurting him. In a few minutes, he told me that his pain was gone. I felt so rewarded – and that I had forged a meaningful connection with a person who would otherwise have remained a stranger!

Not too long after, while visiting at the Crystal Springs Rhododendron Gardens with a friend, she shared with me that she was suffering with the pain of a strained elbow. Again, I was able to quickly alleviate her pain. And have the satisfaction of her relief.

Not that my abilities to channel Reiki were always fool proof in enacting cures. Over the years I have learned that Reiki is a complementary form of treatment that in the case of serious illness should always accompany other medical interventions. Reiki usually does have some type of healing effect, making clients feel more relaxed and comfortable. However, it cannot be relied upon by itself to cure a serious condition.

But early on in my practice I was not as knowledgeable about Reiki's limitations – or as experienced with people's sometimes unrealistic expectations, usually fueled by desperation. And I had yet to develop boundaries or much self-assertiveness. For example, an acquaintance asked me to work on her teenaged, developmentally delayed daughter who was in a late stage of Cancer. As a Reiki 2 practitioner collecting experience, I offered the treatment free of charge. At the end of our session, the daughter, deeply relaxed, needed more downtime. Resting afterwards is always part of the Reiki cure: Reiki enables the body to heal itself, which requires taking it easy. The mother impatiently barked at her dying daughter to "get moving" immediately after the session and and lashed out at me for not curing her daughter of Cancer with one free Reiki session.

Along with expanding in my healing abilities, I have had to learn to manage people's expectations, especially people expecting Reiki to be a miracle cure at the end of a tragic trajectory.

Chery's suggestion to practice at every opportunity included self-practice as well.

I must admit in the early days as a Reiki practitioner I was remiss at practicing Reiki on myself daily as ordered by the Usui Reiki School. (In recent years, I find it increasingly natural to practice daily, an activity which along with the reports of my clients endows me with an unshakeable belief in Reiki's efficacy.) The ability to experience Self Reiki as a newbie did put me into a different relationship with my body – and with life itself. It provided me with a sense of Agency in my ability to achieve physical Well Being and to regulate my emotions when encountering challenges.

During the time I was actively ill with Multiple Chemical Sensitivity (MCS), I was a victim to my body's unpredictable reactions. I could make plans, but the only certainty was that they would sometimes be upset. Once I learned to do Reiki, I had a way to intervene when I was starting to feel ill. This removed my feelings of victimhood and being betrayed by my body.

I'll never forget one of the first times Reiki allowed me to interrupt the progression of my symptoms. It was at an Art of Living Yoga Retreat when I was first starting to travel again. The retreat was in California in February – a perfect time to get away from Portland in the middle of the long rainy season. The retreat setting offered the opportunity to enjoy the outdoors punctuated by a number of indoor activities engaging to the typical Spiritual Seeker, including singing bhajans, instruction in profound and practical Yogic Practices, and talks on Spiritual and Worldly Matters by the Guru Sri Sri Ravi Shankar.

I was getting ready to attend an activity that I had been looking forward to when nausea overcame me. I wasn't sure if I was going to be able to go. I lay down and put my hand on my stomach and was amazed to find in a few minutes time that my stomach problem had evaporated.

The ability to effect change in my state of being made me feel much more hopeful about life. I became convinced of the importance of being in tune with my body. Previously I often blocked my body's signals until they became so overwhelming I had to succumb to illness. Now there were options to exercise. And I now had the ability to make plans - and follow through!

Chapter 10

Over the next 20 years or so leading up to the present, I would expand in my practice of Reiki. Reiki became an important component of my toolbox as I endeavored to live an increasingly normal, productive, and meaningful life. Upon reflection, I understand that Reiki had a stronger influence on me than I gave it credit for at the time. Though consciously my focus was directed externally, Reiki was enabling me to build an inner-directed spiritual foundation that I had been sorely missing in my earlier life. Reiki allowed me to acknowledge my truth and to become increasingly familiar with my inner self through regular communication (i.e., meditation, journaling, and just being present with myself). Increasingly I have become able to rely upon my intuition and find answers to life's difficulties from within myself and through the answers I receive while meditating. And to withstand stress and regulate my emotions when encountering life's ups and downs.

Not too long after I took my Reiki training, I experienced a horrific car accident. It was not my first. I was not "at fault" in this or prior accidents, but I had to acknowledge that some energy I was emitting was causing me to be a magnet for out-of-control drivers.

This car accident was by far the worst. Driving on the I5 freeway from Southwest Portland to my home in North Portland, a long-haul truck drove too close to me and engaged with the side of my car. My car spun around several times; I left my body and found myself elevated to another dimension. There I met my Art of Living guru, Sri Sri Ravi Shankar, who calmed me. Eventually my car stopped spinning. Fortunately, no other cars became involved in the accident on the semi-occupied highway. The cars so easily could have, but instead they bypassed the collision. I was protected from further – and possibly deadly - damage.

I sustained a minor concussion along with back and neck injuries. I was also traumatized, evidenced by the fact that the thought of driving on any highway frankly terrified me for a long time to come – and actually still does. These impairments enabled me to take a leave from the unpleasant and stressful corporate technical writing job at which I had recently begun working (and ultimately enabled me not to return). Fortunately, this was a fulltime permanent job with benefits, a rarity in my work history, so I qualified for short-term disability payments.

Providentially, one of my co-workers, Tanya, was a Reiki practitioner. Through her, I met a Master Reiki practitioner, Marilyn Powers, who would come to influence me greatly as a healer and through the wisdom she imparted for years to come. During the first week after the accident, Tanya and Marilyn gifted me with daily Reiki sessions.

I am convinced that the Reiki they so generously provided made it possible for me to embark upon my healing journey and be restored increasingly to wholeness. Their example also provided me with motivation to make Reiki available at an affordable price – sometimes for free – to those in need.

Over the next twenty years or so, my physical and mental health continued to radically improve. I fulfilled goals and garnered achievements in the outer world that I never thought I'd experience when my health was at its worst. At the low point of my illness, I did not expect to be able to read again, to engage in activities in public, or travel locally let alone internationally. As it turned out, due to my recovery I was able to:

- Continue my jazz singing and band leading, eventually getting paid musical gigs and putting on educational musical events.
- Earn a PhD in Computing Technology in Education, publishing numerous papers and giving talks at many academic conferences all over the world.

- Move to South Korea to teach Digital Media at two universities for a total of five years. This gave me the opportunity to further achieve my life-long goal of world travel and to pursue my research interests. This move also enabled me to be near my son who had moved to South Korea earlier to teach. I continued to travel to give talks at conferences worldwide.

I placed my Reiki practice on the backburner for the first few years of my international travels, but retrieved it to treat a South Korean friend. She was in a great deal of pain resulting from a colonoscopy. The Reiki treatment was effective, evaporating her pain quickly. For the first time, I felt the desire to become a Reiki Master so that I could teach others in South Korea. I felt that Reiki was desperately needed in South Korea, often a harsh and competitive place to live. When I returned to Oregon that summer during break, I worked with my master Chery Esau to earn the Master level of Reiki.

At the age of 61, when my first South Korean university 3-year contract was over, I was at odds about what to do next with my life. My yoga instructor in Seoul recommended that I visit the Indian Yoga Center, Kaivalydham, where she had trained, and where a junior yoga instructor, Sophie Lee, with whom I felt a special connection, was completing her training. Traveling to India had been another one of my life-time goals. Regular breathing and asana practice, along with meditation instruction by spiritual masters at Kaivalydham, impacted me postively as did my other travels in India.

While visiting Benares, I fell while walking by the Ganges River. I did not realize the extent of my injury until later in the day. In the middle of the first segment of a plane trip to Nepal (to where I was traveling to extend my Indian visa) I discovered that I was unable to walk. The kind Australian people around me informed the airplane personnel that

I would need a wheel chair to get me to my next plane. When I arrived in Kathmandu, at the hotel I met a kind and generous lady from Singapore, Jennifer Kwan, who has become a life-long friend, who insisted on taking me to a very skilled body worker the next day. Amazingly, in one session he restored me to normal functioning. I began to contemplate whether the universe was more worthy of trust than I had previously given it credit for. I came to the realization that without effort on my part, the universe had conspired to meet my needs –a new perception for me!

While in India, I procured a position at a different South Korean university for two years. So after my 6-month sojourn, I returned to South Korea for another two years to teach ESL through the arts, including Music and Digital Storytelling. Despite the fact that this university was much less prestigious and well paying than the first, this was some of the most rewarding teaching I had ever done. Then the needs of the university changed and it could no longer use my services as a PhD – and allow me to comply with Visa requirements.

When I returned to the USA at 64 years of age, I was unable to find work. I decided to explore the museum field to see if my digital media education skills might transfer there. I applied for, and garnered, a fellowship as a senior researcher at a prestigious museum complex where I initiated and led an interesting research project. But I did not find the possibility for continuing work. At the finish of the fellowship, I moved back to Portland with no better employment results.

After all I had invested in my career and education, aging out of the USA workforce (where I had never fit easily) was demoralizing. But my increasing ability to help others through Reiki provided confirmation that I still had something to contribute to the world. While I wasn't paying attention, I had become an Elder. My Reiki powers had undeniably grown. After my stint at the Smithsonian, I visited a friend whose dog was limping. After I gave him a treatment, he recovered and she was able to cancel the appointment she had made with the vet. My friend was also having back trouble; the next time she saw the chiropractor after I gave her a treatment, the chiropractor noticed and remarked on the improvement in her spine.

But since I could not find work in the USA, I knew that I would have to relocate elsewhere to survive on the small social security check that I was now eligible for at 65. I researched countries where my $1100 + monthly check would allow me to live and made an exploratory trip to two options: Ecuador and Peru.

The first day that I was in Cuenca, Ecuador, I connected with an organization with which I could offer Reiki. After moving there, I began to establish an in-person Reiki practice.

When the pandemic hit a few months later, I began to work on people via distance. I would come to forge a new profession where my intuitive skills and spiritual capacities, previously on the sidelines, began to emerge into the foreground.

Though the restriction of movement was not easy to contend with (initially Ecuador imposed stringent pandemic lockdowns), I found that my inner landscape was for the most part tranquil. I did not have a robust support system in Cuenca, but I did have several USA friends as well as my son in Japan, with whom I was regularly in touch via technology. This social contact greatly helped my mental health. But I also found that much more than in my earlier life, I could rely on my own counsel - and myself.

Chapter 11

A friend and former distance Reiki patient recently died. I was devastated by her passing. Although she shared with me that she was terminal, her death occurred much earlier than anticipated. We had been speaking regularly prior to her passing, but once her cancer commenced, with the simultaneous weakening of her voice as well as her body, she halted our regular communications. Eventually she began to employ me to do distance Reiki on her on a monthly basis, not with the goal of curing her cancer but to ease her transition and make her more comfortable. We did, however, have one last phone call prior to the last distance Reiki session – which neither of us knew would be the last.

She told me about a trip from which she had recently returned and the old friends and sights with which she had reconnected. She had asked me to prepare her for it with a Reiki session because she had felt discomfort before leaving, and she did not want her pain to hamper her enjoyment of her trip too much. She recounted that a number of mishaps did occur on her journey, including problems with the car, pain when standing, and difficulty with doing much walking. She told me she felt especially connected to me because of the distance Reiki I had been sending her – she strongly felt the bond of the sharing.

I found the aftermath of our last session – which occurred right after the phone call – deeply unsettling. I focused on her requests: to send Reiki to the tumors in her abdomen that were affecting her left shoulder blade, to her left side and lower back, and to address her tiredness, lack of energy, and her stress from the situation and the ambiguity of her future.

While I was sending the Reiki, the energy felt discordant. It surprised me because that was unusual. The energy was not exactly painful, but not comforting and pleasant as usual. I remembered experiencing this energy as a patient once and being repelled by the sensation. Also –

when the session ended, the sending energy halted abruptly. I always end the session when the energy I am channeling ceases, but in this case the boundary between the presence of energy and its absence was more marked.

I would learn that within a day she was experiencing such disabling pain that she was again in the hospital. We had several brief interchanges in the interlude between our phone conversation and her death. I was of course horrified to think that the Reiki I had administered was in any way responsible for the pain she was experiencing and her swift demise. She asked me if there was anything unusual about our Reiki session, and I told her about the discordant energy I experienced and the extremely abrupt cessation of the energy at the end of the session.

I know I did not do anything purposefully to hurt her – I loved this person! – but to be truthful this experience made me think twice about my willingness to engage in Reiki with the terminally ill, to offer myself as a channel for energies over which I have no control.

I was stunned to read her husband's Facebook post saying that she had transitioned less than two weeks after our last phone call and Reiki session. I was aware that she was dying, but during our last phone call she informed me that she was thinking of moving to another city where she might be able to receive better care - and perhaps a cure. In our shared reality, we both figured that she'd be around for at least a year – she had new projects she wanted to begin during her remaining time! I followed up our phone conversation by contacting an old friend, a video editor, to see if she would be willing to help Elizabeth with a video project she was wanting to post on YouTube about her experience with Cancer and death.

Also during our last phone conversation, ever the giver, Elizabeth gave me several excellent pieces of advice and some connections to help me further my career. We were both thinking about the future, but as it turned out, I was the one who would be continuing on the earth plane.

I found it very hard to cope with the feelings I had about Elizabeth's death. After learning she had transitioned, I was overcome with feelings of sorrow. Worried that I would be bad company, I considered cancelling a lunch date with a new acquaintance. Concluding that the distraction might do me some good, I decided to go nonetheless. Among the new places I had not yet experienced, Diane took me to a marketplace where indigenous women were offering spiritual cleansings, known as limpiezas. I decided I could use one.

As the Ecuadorian healer worked on me, I experienced waves of grief. Although uncomfortable, it was also good to be able to access these feelings that I had been cut off from. When the healer finished, she told me that I was experiencing fear and nervousness. Not unusual, I concluded, for someone who had just experienced the death of someone close - that she felt she might have contributed to!

Later on when I was alone, I felt a connection with Elizabeth. Through my intuition I heard her tell me that she was there and would be available even though she had moved to another dimension. I also understood that she would be reincarnating soon into another being for whom it would be much easier to accomplish the visionary goals she had been anxious to implement.

Later that night, before I went to sleep, I noticed a globe of light on my ceiling within which some movement was occurring. I assumed that this meant she was hatching into another dimension as a different being. The next night, the globe of light appeared again as a pure burst of light. The third night after my emotions were more settled, through the acupressure points I had pressed and the yogic breathing I had practiced, the globe of light did not appear.

Chapter 12

The ability to access different dimensions is something I have acquired unconsciously over the years as my spiritual skills have increased. Over the last 20 years, I had slowly grown a connection with Source and my inner guidance system. Learning to breathe and meditate played a big part. This has made it possible for me to regulate my emotions in difficult circumstances. It provided me with courage and enabled me to receive guidance enabling me to follow an unconventional path necessary for my survival.

Many experiences during this time taught me the importance of self-care, listening to one's body, and heeding one's intuition. They included the healings I received from my teachers Marilyn Powers and Chery Esau, the Reiki sessions I gave myself and others, and my participation in Yoga practices, community music, and Rick Hanson's Foundations of Well Being program. As I achieved inner equilibrium through these practices, I was better able to connect with myself and to receive messages from Source. I learned to put myself at the center of my universe rather than seeking to fit in. I learned to assume my power and agency to move out of victim consciousness.

Because of my own healing, I am in a psychological place a good deal of the time where I am vibrating at a pretty harmonious level. When I prepare to do Reiki - especially at a distance, I engage in meditative techniques that allow me to raise my energy stream even higher. In person, the Reiki flows naturally.

Reiki operates on the principle that people's energy streams entrain with each other, with the higher influencing the lower to elevate. As a Reiki practitioner I create a Reiki space in person or via distance with energy vibrating higher than my normal. When I practice Reiki, I share this energy stream with others, lifting them up and restoring them.

Additionally, when working by distance, I am provided with restorative visualizations – like movies - that I transmit.

According to Edgar Cayce, the human body contains interfaces with spiritual and mental dimensions of reality, existing within the glandular and nervous systems. Throughout my life, I have been able to tune into frequencies outside of the body/mind. The gradual growth of my telepathic ability to plug into the universal web has enabled me to establish a connection to treat over distances. After entering into a semi-trance state with the aid of binaural beats, I intuitively know how to transmit energy to treat a client's body and mind via distance, receiving visualizations and movies to heal the client physically and psychologically.

As I have progressed in my Reiki journey, a major result is the ability to connect to other beings including animals. On several occasions within the last year I have been amazed by my affectionate reception by animals that I have run across in chance encounters. This includes a horse I met while on a hike, a llama I met on a tour, and a dog who clamored to a sidewalk to safety after receiving a telepathic message from me to depart from the center of the busy street. Earlier in my life I suffered from terrible social anxiety, but lately I feel pretty much at home wherever I go even if I do not feel strongly attuned to the people – or animals - I find there.

Ultimately an effect of progress in the Reiki Journey is to feel strongly connected with oneself, one's inner voice, and to be able to connect with Source for guidance when in doubt. Reiki allows one to transcend fear and to be truthful with oneself. It engenders trust in life and cultivates the ability to focus – and to be in the Now.

Chapter 13

They say as people age they become happier with their lives, even if objectively there is not so much to be happy about in terms of money, status, and definitely not looks and bodily functioning. It is an ironic, although lucky, thing that as others value us less, we finally come to value ourselves more. Reiki can help with this self-valuing.

In my case, not only am I benefitting from this state of affairs at the age of 71, but additionally from the effects of Reiki and my Reiki Practice and an undeniable increase in my Reiki abilities.

Aging comes with a number of physical changes – and developmental stages – that we are often not prepared for. Although we may think we are familiar enough with the elderly around us, the experience of aging can ambush us when we go through it ourselves.

In my case, upon returning from university teaching abroad, finding I had aged out of the USA workforce came as a shock. Despite my advanced education and many years of work experience, I had no way to earn a living. I similarly found myself out in the cold when I strove to participate in the jazz activities in which for years I had developed expertise and been enthusiastically involved.

As a female senior I discovered there was no role for me in the USA except that of a consumer. The money I had to live on – a pittance of a Social Security check - was not enough to afford me a dignified way of life in the USA.

I ended up moved to Ecuador – a welcoming country where I could afford to live. In the move, I discarded a lot that I did not have the means to bring: possessions and preoccupations. But I was grateful to be in Ecuador and to have the opportunity in my third age to consciously forge a new and different life, one far more aligned with my true self.

People often ask me how I came upon the decision to leave the USA and how I found the courage to move. I attribute it to preplanning and research – and the transformation I experienced through Reiki.

I had been thinking about retirement for many years. After my lengthy recovery from my workplace poisoning, for which I had never been compensated, I went back to school to get a doctorate hoping that would put me in a position to find lucrative employment after years working in the gig economy. As a 50 plus PhD, the only higher education work I could find was overseas. While culturally enriching, the pay was not. I accepted that despite my best efforts, circumstances - including my health challenges - had conspired to obstruct amassing the resources to have a comfortable USA retirement.

Because I traveled widely and had spent a number of years living abroad, I was open to the possibility of relocating in retirement. My son – who was also living an international life – had repeatedly encouraged me to consider foreign options. So when the time came that I was forced into retirement after relentlessly and unsuccessfully pursuing options for work in the USA, I accepted reality and with boots on the ground explored the possibilities open to me with my finances – which at that time were Ecuador and Peru. I chose Ecuador because I could obtain a professional visa there allowing me to work whereas I understood that in Peru I would not be able to work for several years.

How did Reiki assist me with this major life challenge? Reiki gave me a clear mind, removing the depression and anxiety I had experienced in my younger days. Reiki practice helped me to recognize reality and to accept and support myself when the external world was not reflecting this acceptance back to me. Reiki relieved my stress and helped me to regulate my emotions so that I could view my travels in the pursuit of a new domicile as an exciting adventure and not be crippled by anger, bitterness and disappointment at my plight. Reiki gave me confidence that I would be up to coping with any threats that might arise – and believe me, some did! – and have the moxie to diffuse them. Reiki gifted me with the empowerment to take responsibility for my own situation and to find my own solution.

In **Wise Aging: Living with Joy, Resilience and Spirit**, Rabbi Rachel Cowan and Dr. Linda Thai discuss the opportunities and challenges that can come with age. The development of aspects of inner consciousness including focus, a strong kinesthetic connection with one's own body or "feeling sense", and the cultivation of non-local awareness can be positive features of this time of life. Challenges include a transformed relationship to physicality; the need for agency in healthcare, including self care; and staying connected - and finding new ways to be of value - to friends and family as well as the world at large. And, of course, coming to grips with death is another quandary whose resolution can result in considerable peace.

My Reiki practice has accompanied and supported me as I have grappled, and gained some mastery, of all of these issues. As a Reiki practitioner, the development of inner consciousness has exponentially upgraded my healing capabilities. Focusing on myself rather than attempting to control others has greatly enhanced my relationships with friends and family members. Offering my Reiki skills to others in need – particularly young Ecuadorian people – has helped me to bridge differences and strengthen my relationships with others in the community with whom I might otherwise not connect. I have had a major health issue to cope with recently along with the inevitable – but unforeseen - physical changes that accompany age. The self-acceptance and self-trust engendered by Reiki has helped me to confront and conquer these physical challenges with some equanimity.

And so I advocate Reiki as a helpful resource for all seniors, not just as receivers but as practitioners at any level from Reiki 1 to Reiki Master.

While as clients they can experience the soothing of pains and lessening of stress and anxiety that often accompany aging, as Reiki practitioners, seniors can do this for themselves - as well as for friends and family - at any time of their choosing. And they can experience the unique transformation and empowerment especially beneficial for Elders navigating the challenges intrinsic to this time of life.

.

Epilogue

Not only does Reiki provide many attributes necessary for successful aging but also cultivates many of the qualities necessary for artistry, whether as a storyteller of film and drama or a performing artist: an actor, vocalist, or instrumentalist. I have been an artist of one fashion or another throughout my life, and in my later years have enjoyed assisting others as an educator in pursuing their own creativity. Reiki engenders the self-trust and bravery necessary to embark upon the creative journey. And as I have experienced, involvement in the expressive arts can ignite healing in individuals.

I have decided in the next phase of my career to explore and transmit methods to integrate Reiki not only with aging but also with the expressive arts. Identifying myself to the public to do this work requires being "out" as an intuitive. While I spent my earlier professional life being largely closeted about my metaphysical interests, in giving myself the gift of finally expressing my entire self in my work, I must introduce myself to the public in my entirety: a person who believes that not everything is visible and material. One who is firmly convinced that energy constitutes all of life.

I can now accept that being honest about my beliefs may cause some people to reject me. In my younger days, I would have found this rejection extremely painful – in addition to fearing that it would affect my livelihood. But today the world has changed as have my circumstances. I recognize the positives of being truly oneself and look forward to the adventures that lie ahead!

Don't miss out!

Visit the website below and you can sign up to receive emails whenever Sunny Cohen publishes a new book. There's no charge and no obligation.

https://books2read.com/r/B-A-RHTBB-QDHRC

BOOKS 2 READ

Connecting independent readers to independent writers.

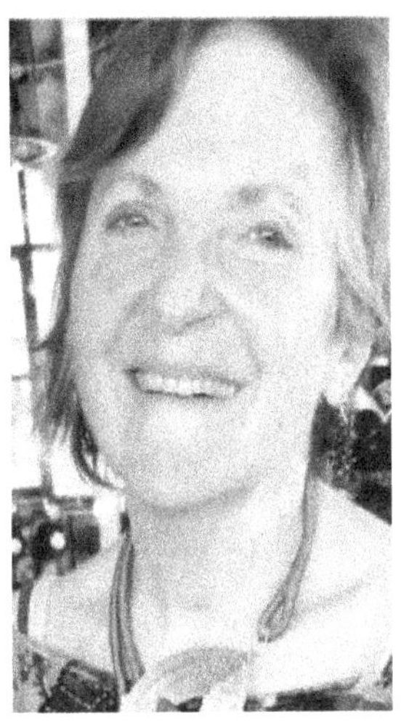

About the Author

During her award winning, internationally recognized career as an educator and artist, author Sunny Cohen simultaneously cultivated a spiritual and intuitive path. Highly intuitive as a child, Sunny has had a life-long interest in metaphysics. A workplace poisoning in the early 90s started Sunny on her path of self healing through Reiki. Now an elder, Sunny has had a wide variety of lived experience in family, work, and political and artistic endeavors and as an empath can relate to many of her clients' life situations. Sunny began studying and practicing Reiki in 1998 and became a Reiki Master in 2011, initiated in the Usui Method by Reiki Master Chery Esau of Portland, Oregon, USA. Upon retiring from her previous work as a professor, researcher and interdisciplinary artist, Reiki became Cohen's main focus in 2017.

Read more at https://www.sunnycohenreiki.org/.

www.ingramcontent.com/pod-product-compliance
Lightning Source LLC
Chambersburg PA
CBHW070317160726
47999CB00003B/1061